BASIC HOME REMEDIES

A MACROBIOTIC GUIDE TO SPECIAL DRINKS, COMPRESSES, PLASTERS, AND OTHER NATURAL APPLICATIONS

BY MICHIO KUSHI
EDITED BY ALEX JACK

ONE PEACEFUL WORLD PRESS
BECKET, MASSACHUSETTS

Diane Hannan

Basic Home Remedies
© 1994 by Michio Kushi and Alex Jack

Published by One Peaceful World Press, Becket, Massachusetts,
U.S.A.

For further information on mail-order sales, wholesale or retail
discounts, distribution, translations, and foreign rights, please
contact the publisher:

One Peaceful World Press
P.O. Box 10
Leland Road
Becket, MA 01223
U.S.A.

Telephone (413) 623–2322
Fax (413) 623-8827

First Edition: May 1994
10 9 8 7 6 5 4 3 2 1

ISBN 1–882984–08–0
Printed in U.S.A.

IMPORTANT NOTICE TO THE READER

The information in this book was presented by Michio Kushi at a special seminar of the Macrobiotic Educators' Association (M.E.A.) for teacher training and development in Becket, Massachusetts, in January, 1994. It represents the most current application of his teachings and includes significant changes, modifications, and innovations from previously published material.

The information and remedies presented in this book are for educational purposes. Their aim is to acquaint the general public with simple, inexpensive, and easy-to-administer home remedies that have been traditionally used and are generally safe. They are meant to complement, not replace, the care and guidance of your physician or other medical professional. If you have any reason to suspect a serious illness or life-threatening disorder, or have had a serious accident, you are strongly advised to seek the advice of a qualified macrobiotic teacher and/or medical diagnosis and attention. There are an increasing number of doctors and other healthcare professionals who are open to integrating traditional home remedies into their treatment, including some of the dietary preparations and external applications described in this book.

RESOURCES

The One Peaceful World Society was founded by Michio Kushi as an international information network and friendship society of individuals, families, educational centers, organic farmers, teachers, parents and children, authors and artists, homemakers and businesspeople, and others devoted to the realization of a healthy, peaceful world. Activities include educational and spiritual tours, international food aid, and publishing and communications. Membership is $30/year for individuals and $50/year for families. Benefits include the quarterly *One Peaceful World Newsletter* and a free book from OPW Press. To join or obtain more information, please contact:

> One Peaceful World
> P.O. Box 10, Leland Road
> Becket, MA 01223, U.S.A.
> Telephone (413) 623-2322
> Fax (413) 623-8827

The Kushi Institute is an educational center for macrobotic and holistic studies located in the Berkshire mountains of western Massachusetts with affiliates in Europe and extention programs in selected cities in the United States and Canada. Programs include the weekly Way to Health Program (offering classes in home remedy preparation and cooking), Michio Kushi Seminars, and Dynamics of Macrobiotics. For information, contact:

> Kushi Institute
> P.O. Box 7, Leland Road
> Becket, MA 01223, U.S.A.
> Telephone (413) 623-5741
> Fax (413) 623-8827

INTRODUCTION

The preparations and techniques presented in this book are based upon traditional home remedies that have been used for thousands of years. They also include a variety of new drinks, compresses, and plasters that I have developed over the last thirty years to deal with the common conditions and disorders of modern society—such as hypoglycemia—that were rare in the past. They are an important part of macrobiotics, a way of life based on understanding natural order and creating health, especially through the proper selection and preparation of whole, natural foods.

Modern medicine has many wonderful dimensions, including effective diagnosis, emergency care, and reduction of pain. But some drugs and procedures are potentially dangerous, expensive, difficult to administer, and have harmful side effects. The basic home cares presented in this book are simple, safe, inexpensive, and efficient. Unless incorrectly prepared or administered for the wrong reason, they do not produce undesirable side effects, nor are they harmful to the environment. (A high percentage of modern drugs originate from the tropical rain forests and have a destructive effect on the planet's delicate ecosystem.) They are also easy to prepare and bring medicine back into the reach of the family. They do not require a large medical or pharmaceutical staff.

Traditional medicine was based on yin/yang thinking—or the balance of complementary opposites—and an energetic understanding of healing. In treating various conditions, substances were selected that had a complementary/opposite energy (for example, the use of plants to treat human beings). Moreover, foods that had a similar look or shape were fitted to particular organs. Thus for lung troubles, lotus root which had the shape of the alveoli of the lungs was recommended. For the pancreas, which has a more round structure, cabbage and onions were used. To repel worms in the intestines, which resemble the ancient ocean in which life began, a wormlike sea vegetable known as Corsican Tea was traditionally taken.

Another yin/yang principle is to include a little of the opposite energy in a home remedy. Take a classroom of boys, for example. To stimulate them, the best way is to bring in a girl. Then everything is more highly charged. The same way, to activate a group of girls, bring in a boy. With special drinks, compresses, and plasters, we introduce a little of the opposite energy to make the remedy more active. For example, we add a little grated ginger—which gives a yin, dispersing effect—to Ume-Sho-Kuzu Tea that is designed overall to have a slightly more yang, gathering effect.

Our way involves a safe, mild approach. The remedies in this book are recommended only for a short time—from one to three days in many cases, to seven to ten days in other cases, to several months in a few cases. Generally, it is more effective to stop a special drink or compress after a brief time and then let the stimulated organs work and adjust, and then repeat the remedy a few days, a week, or a few weeks later. Also, from the second month, the condition usually improves, so you don't need to take as much. In the proper use of home remedies, less is more. Overuse of remedies—like overeating, even of good quality macrobiotic food—can be a cause of imbalance.

Compared to changing our way of eating, way of thinking, and way of life, home remedies are a symptomatic approach to health. They will temporarily help alleviate certain conditions, but unless the underlying way of life is changed, symptoms will invariably return. Please see my book, *Standard Macrobiotic Diet* (One Peaceful World Press) for an introduction on getting started and the full scope and variety of the macrobiotic way of eating. Still, many remedies such as the ginger compress, are so effective that anyone may benefit from their application, and the experience of such a simple, inexpensive treatment can change a person's way of thinking and stimulate them in a more holistic direction.

It is especially useful to apply these methods when you have just started to eat macrobiotically, as the body's eliminatory processes are more active at this time. In the beginning, as the body adjusts to whole, natural foods, it begins to eliminate excess. We call this process discharging, and in addition to normal eliminatory channels such as the urine and bowel movements, excess may be discharged through fever, coughing, or other abnormal means. Some of the remedies serve to make the discharge process more comfortable or control its frequency and duration. But once again, be careful. In the beginning, it is sometimes difficult to distinguish a worsening condition from a discharge. Please seek the advice and

6

guidance of an experienced macrobiotic teacher and/or medical professional.

After changing to a more healthful way of life, stagnation from past imbalance may remain in the body. Some of the remedies in this book are designed to help discharge old fat and cholesterol deposits from past hamburger, chicken, egg, or dairy food consumption. To erase the most harmful effects of heavy animal food intake takes only several months, but deep blockages will take several years of good eating to release altogether.

When preparing home remedies, it is usually best to take them on an empty stomach, such as mid-morning or mid-afternoon or sometimes in the early evening. However, it is better not to eat or drink three hours before sleeping in order to allow for proper digestion.

Further information on the preparation and proper use of these and other home remedies is available from the Kushi Institute in Becket, Massachusetts, including Personal Educational Sessions with a macrobiotic teacher to discuss individual and family needs.

In preparing this book, I am grateful to Alex Jack for editing; to Edward Esko for reviewing the text; to Gale Jack for copyediting and proofreading; and to the teachers, students, and staff of the Kushi Institute.

The medicine of the future will be a combination of traditional methods and approaches and new techniques and applications that are developed to meet everchanging personal, social, and environmental conditions. Together let us create a New Medicine for Humanity to enable our species to enter the new century safely and continue our natural biological and spiritual evolution for endless generations.

Michio Kushi
March, 1994
Brookline, Massachusetts

AME KUZU TEA

This drink helps relax mind and body. It is especially recommended for children and can bring down fever in small children. It is also good for stomach and intestinal problems, hypoglycemia, premenstrual and menstrual cramps, and tension caused by intake of too much yang such as chips, crackers, and other hard baked goods. In olden days, monks would drink ame kuzu after begging in order to make themselves mellow and relaxed to study.

1. Dissolve one heaping teaspoon of kuzu in two or three tablespoons of cold water.

2. Add one cup cold water to the dissolved kuzu.

3. Add 1-2 teaspoons rice syrup or barley malt, or one-half cup apple juice.

4. Bring to a boil over a medium flame, stirring constantly to avoid lumping, until the liquid becomes translucent. Reduce the flame as low as possible. Drink while hot.

AZUKI BEAN TEA

Azuki beans are small, red beans and are more yang relative to other beans. They are native to Japan and the Far East and are now grown in the United States. For daily cooking, the American variety are fine, but for medicinal use, the Oriental ones are stronger.

Azuki bean tea is good for the regulation of kidney and urinary functions. It helps produce a smooth bowel movement. Kidney troubles are often caused by taking too much dairy food; in this case kombu is more effective to use in seasoning than salt. Otherwise, a pinch of sea salt may be added toward the end of simmering. If no seasoning is added, you may feel a little weak after several days.

To counter recent heavy animal food intake, take 1 small cup of this tea for 3 to 4 days. If constipated, reduce use. To help relieve more chronic conditions, take daily, every other day, or every third day for about 3 weeks depending on the condition.

1. Place one cup of beans in a pot with a two-inch strip of kombu (soaked and finely chopped).

2. Add four cups of water and bring to a boil.

3. Lower the flame, cover and simmer for one-half hour.

4. Strain out the beans and drink the liquid while hot.

Variations: • To help dissolve kidney stones, add one-half cup fresh grated daikon at the end of cooking, after you strain out the beans. Drink the liquid, eat the pulp.

• To relieve mucus in the kidneys or urinary tract, add one-half cup fresh grated lotus root and prepare as in above variation. Lotus root releases any stagnation including mucus created by dairy, sugar, or fat.

• You may make this drink a little yin, especially if taking for several days, by adding a touch of barley malt or rice syrup.

BANCHA DOUCHE

This remedy helps to eliminate stagnated mucus and fat in the region of the uterus and vagina.

1. Use one quart bancha tea, cooled to body temperature.

2. Add one three-finger pinch of sea salt plus one teaspoon of brown rice vinegar.

3. Stir all together, pour into douche bag, and douche after a Daikon Hip Bath.

BLACK SOYBEAN TEA

Black Soybean Tea is good for loosening, softening, and warming up. It gives a relaxing effect and is more yin than azuki bean tea. In Japan, it is traditionally made for New Year's. With long-time cooking, the soybeans become very sweet, so a sweet taste is not customarily added to this drink.

This tea is good for kidney, bladder, and reproductive problems, especially yang troubles caused by an accumulation of fat. These include cramping, heavy menstruation, or constipation from animal food intake. It is also good for promoting mother's milk, especially when cooked with mochi. Black Soybean Tea is also very good for some coughs, especially yang, dry coughs, and for laryngitis.

For less acute symptoms, it is generally taken 2 to 3 times a week. For acute ones, a cup may be taken daily. Sea salt may be added at the end of cooking for seasoning instead of kombu. For more yang people, however, it is better to use no seasoning.

1.   Place one cup of black soybeans in a pot with a two-inch strip of dry kombu (soaked and finely chopped).

2.   Add four cups of water and bring to a boil.

3.   Lower the flame and simmer for 30 to 45 minutes.

4.   Strain the beans from the water.

5.   Drink this dark, slightly sweet liquid while hot.

6.   You may continue cooking the beans longer until soft and edible.

Variation: • Add one-half cup dried daikon to preparation from the beginning. Strain the vegetables with the beans.

• Adding 25 percent daikon, and 25 percent lotus, and a little shiitake mushroom is helpful for breast tumors caused by cheese and other animal food.

BODY SCRUB

The body scrub helps activate circulation and better energy flow through the entire body. It helps to discharge fat accumulated under the skin and open pores to promote smooth and regular elimination of any excess fat and toxins. It also promotes clean, clear skin. The body scrub can be done once or twice daily, in the morning and/or at night, before or after a shower or bath, but apart from it.

1. Dip a small cotton towel or cloth in hot water. Wring out the excess water.

2. Scrub the whole body, dipping the towel or cloth into hot water again when cool. Be sure to include the hands and feet and each finger and toe.

3. The skin should become pink or slightly red. This result may take a few days to achieve, if the skin is clogged with accumulated fats.

BROWN RICE/MISO PLASTER

For centuries, miso—fermented soybean paste—has been used in the Far East as a plaster to heal skin infections and allergic conditions, as well as radiation or fire burns and simple cuts (see Miso Plaster). If the area is red and irritated, a plaster containing miso is good to heal and prevent infectious conditions. However, if the skin is ruptured, don't apply.

The salt in the miso causes the affected area to shrink. By adding 50 percent brown rice to the plaster, the shrinking is reduced. The rice further serves to calm and soothe the region. Together the rice and miso soften, as in the case of hard tumors, make the skin smooth and prevent infection, and cool down, as in the case of burns or radiation exposure. This plaster can also be applied for muscle tension or tissue tension. The area will become soft, smooth, and flexible. This plaster may also be used for bruises, broken bones, and accidents.

1. Use softly cooked, unsalted brown rice (cooled to room temperature) and mash well in a suribachi.

2. Mix with an equal amount of miso.

3. Add 3-4 percent grated ginger and mix together thoroughly, adding a small amount of water to make into a soft plaster.

4. Spread this mixture from one-half to one inch thickness on a cotton cloth.

5. Apply the mixture directly to the skin (not the cloth side) and leave on for one to two hours, or three hours or longer in some cases. Secure in place with a bandage or tie with a cotton strip, if necessary. The plaster is effective until half dry.

BUCKWHEAT PLASTER

The Buckwheat Plaster is a traditional Far Eastern remedy to help draw out water or other excess fluids that are retained by the body. It may be applied to swollen areas on the legs, arms, abdomen, etc.

Buckwheat, which is a very yang, grainlike plant, attracts and draws out the more yin water or liquid. It is more effective to make fresh flour from whole buckwheat groats than to use packaged buckwheat flour. The energy is much stronger; however, if groats are not available, you may use store-bought flour.

Apply first a Hot Towel Compress or Ginger Compress to the affected region to make the area hot before applying the Buckwheat Plaster. The plaster should be as stiff, hot, and dry as possible.

1. Mix buckwheat flour with a little sesame oil and enough hot water to form a stiff, hard dough.

2. Spread the dough on a cotton cloth, about three-quarters of an inch thick.

3. Apply the dough side (not the cloth side) directly to the swollen area.

4. Remove after one to two hours.

5. As the plaster draws out the fluid, the dough will become soft and watery. When this happens, replace the plaster with a new, stiff dough.

CARROT/DAIKON DRINK

I first developed this drink for liver troubles, to help discharge eggs, cheese, and beef fat. But this preparation is helpful in dissolving fat deposits anywhere within the body and quickly reducing high cholesterol. It also helps dissolve calcified stones in such areas as kidneys and gall bladder. I now recommend it for many chronic conditions, including many forms of heart disease and tumors.

Daikon is more yin and gives a dissolving effect. Carrot is more yang and is added to strengthen and help move energy down in the body. However, if continuously taken together they weaken. By adding the umeboshi and nori, this drink can be taken for a relatively long time: every day for 10 days or every other day for 3 weeks.

1. Finely grate one-half cup each of carrots and daikon. Place in a saucepan. Don't let the gratings sit for a long time.

2. Add two cups of water and bring to a gentle boil.

3. Add one-third of a sheet of nori and one-half of an umeboshi plum, cooked together with the grated vegetables.

4. Simmer for about 3 minutes and add a few drops of shoyu/soy sauce toward the end.

5. Eat and drink the vegetables and the broth.

Variation: • Add one-third cup of grated lotus root, especially for lung or lymphatic conditions. A little scallion or ginger may be added to the basic recipe if desired.

CHLOROPHYLL (LEAFY GREENS) PLASTER

The leaves of large, leafy green vegetables are very helpful in cooling down fever, neutralizing inflammation, and relieving burns and bruises. Sometimes just putting leaves (either big ones or ones that grow upward) such as cabbage leaves, collard greens, turnip tops, or daikon tops on the head, chest, or arms will provide immediate relief. Cabbage is particularly good because it is a more yang vegetable and has drawing, or contractive, power. The Chlorophyll Plaster has a more concentrated effect and may be used directly or after whole leaves have absorbed the initial heat.

1. Finely chop several green leafy vegetables such as daikon leaves, kale, collards, cabbage, Chinese cabbage, etc.

2. Place in a suribachi and mash well.

3 Add 10-20 percent unbleached white flour and mix into a paste.

4. Spread the mixture about one-half inch thick on a towel or cloth and apply the greens directly to the skin (not the cloth side). Leave on for two to three hours.

CORSICAN TEA

This tea made from Corsican seaweed is traditionally known as *Makuri* and is taken in the Far East to prevent or relieve intestinal worms. Japanese children customarily received a cup of this tea at school.

Eating raw salad can lead to worms in the body, and organic vegetables sometimes contain worm eggs. Also worms are found in all sorts of animal food, including fish. According to Oriental diagnosis, biting the fingernails is a sign that worms are nibbling in the body.

The tea is smelly, strong tasting, and looks something like worms. But it effectively kills round worms and pin worms and their eggs and flushes out the intestinal tract. It is also good for women's troubles, such as weakness after childbirth.

Corsican Tea should be taken on an empty stomach. Skip breakfast and take one big cup at lunchtime. Then the worms will become intoxicated and come out.

1. Prepare a handful of Corsican seaweed in 4 to 6 cups of water, bring to a boil, and let simmer for about 20 minutes.

2. Take daily for 3 to 5 days; wait about a week; and then repeat.

Variation: • Another traditional treatment for worms is to skip breakfast and lunch. Then when hungry, eat a handful of raw rice (let it soak in your mouth before chewing), along with half a handful of raw pumpkin or sunflower seeds, and a half handful of raw scallion, onion, or garlic. Wait two hours before having a regular meal. Do this for 3 days in a row, then wait 7 to 10 days, and do again for 3 days.

DAIKON DRINK NO. 1

This tea will help to lower fevers by inducing sweat. It brings relief from food poisoning caused by meat, fish or shellfish. It promotes sweating and opens up people who have been eating dairy food or whose condition is overly yang.

1. Grate about three tablespoons of fresh daikon.

2. Mix the daikon with one-quarter teaspoon grated ginger and a few drops of shoyu/soy sauce.

3. Pour two or three cups of hot bancha-twig tea or stem tea over the mixed ingredients.

4. Drink as much of the tea as possible while hot.

5. After drinking this tea, go to bed and wrap yourself in a blanket to induce perspiration.

Note:
• **Since this tea is very strong, do not take more than twice a day for one or two days.**

• For children, limit the quantity to one-half cup per day.

• To reduce fever in babies and young children, it is better to give apple juice, grated apple or a kuzu drink with rice syrup (see Ame Kuzu Tea).

DAIKON DRINK NO. 2

This drink induces urination and relieves swollen ankles and feet.

1. Grate one-half cup of daikon.

2. Place daikon in a cheesecloth and squeeze out the juice.

3. To two tablespoons of juice, add six tablespoons of water.

4. Bring to a boil, reduce the flame, and allow to simmer gently for a maximum of one minute.

5. Add a pinch of sea salt or a few drops of shoyu/soy sauce toward the end of cooking.

6. Drink this preparation once each day or once every two days, for no more than three times in a row.

With dried daikon:

1. Add one-half cup of dried daikon to two and one-half cups fresh, cold water.

2. Bring to a gentle boil. Cover then lower the flame.

3. Simmer 20 minutes then strain out the vegetables.

4. Drink this broth while hot, warm, or at room temperature.

5. You may add the leftover dried daikon to other vegetable dishes.

Variations:
- Add one shiitake mushroom and prepare as above.

- Or add 1-2 inches of dry kombu sea vegetable and prepare as above.

DAIKON HIP BATH

This treatment warms the body; is good for women's reproductive organs and for skin problems; aids in extracting body odors due to the consumption of animal foods; and draws out excess fat and oil from the body.

1. Dry fresh daikon leaves in a shady place until they are brown and brittle. If daikon leaves are not available, use turnip leaves or a handful of arame sea vegetable.

2. Place about four to five bunches of dried leaves or a handful of arame in a large pot.

3. Add four to five quarts of water and bring to a boil.

4. Reduce to a medium flame and simmer until water is brown.

5. Add approximately one cup of any kind of sea salt to the pot and stir well to dissolve.

6. Pour the hot liquid into a small tub or bath. Add water until the bath level is waist-high when sitting in the tub.

7. Keep the temperature as hot as possible and cover your upper body with a large towel to induce perspiration.

8. Stay in the bath for 10 to 20 minutes or until the hip becomes very red and hot.

9. Keep this hip area warm after coming out of the bath.

10. This bath is best and most effective just before bedtime, but at least an hour after eating.

Variation: If daikon or other leaves or arame is not available, do a Salt Hip Bath, following the process outlined above, using a handful or any kind of sea salt in the hot bath water.

21

DAIKON PLASTER

In the Orient, daikon is the most popular vegetable used in cooking, pickling, and in medicinal preparations. The leaves and root are customarily used. In the early days of macrobiotics in Boston, we got seeds from Japan and gave them to New England farmers. That was the beginning of daikon growing in America.

The purpose of the Daikon Plaster is to dissolve hard animal fat on the periphery of the body such as chicken fat, dairy fat, or anything clogging the capillaries beneath the skin and blocking circulation. It is also good for bruises, surface burns, fevers, inflammations, or swellings. It helps to cool down and to clean up internal bleeding.

Daikon has a pungent, stimulating effect. Use only for a short time until the skin becomes red. Although it begins to irritate if left for too long, the Daikon Plaster is milder than the Mustard Plaster. Because it is pungent, we don't add grated ginger, as with some other plasters. If it becomes too hot, take it off.

The Daikon Plaster is a simple, quick application for local stagnation, to improve blood and energy circulation.

1.   Grate several ounces of daikon. Do not use the juice. Mix with a little flour.

2.   Apply to the bruised or affected area. Leave on for 15 to 30 minutes. For large bruises, repeat several days.

Variation: • Turnip may be substituted if daikon is not available.

DRIED DAIKON TEA

We use daikon in many home remedies. But fresh daikon has a strong yin effect and the person becomes weak after one or two days. Dried daikon is stronger than fresh daikon and can be used for a longer period of time. Several years ago, I introduced Dried Daikon Tea. It is good for dissolving all fatty substances and a small cup can be taken daily for 2 to 3 months.

Dried daikon can be made at home from the roots in your garden or purchased at the natural foods store. Often it is sold shredded in packages imported from Japan. The best dried daikon I've seen is from the Andes Mountain region in South America, and we occasionally have some at the Kushi Foundation Store in Becket.

1. Combine 1 part dried, shredded daikon to 4 parts water.

2. Bring to a boil, reduce flame, and simmer 15-30 minutes.

3. Toward the end of cooking, add a pinch of sea salt and let simmer until done.

Notes: • This drink is good for headaches in the back or sides of the head and migraines. For ear problems, give this drink and a Ginger Compress on the kidney and ear. It can be used after delivery by mothers whose infants are jaundiced.

Variations: • The standard method of seasoning is with a pinch of salt or small piece of kombu. For liver/ gallbladder conditions, you may use umeboshi plum instead. For lung or liver conditions, use shiso leaves, and for lungs add lotus root. A weak person needs seasoning with this drink or the tea makes them too weak. The drink is already yin, so don't add sweetener.

• This tea is often prepared with lotus root, shiitake mushroom, and kombu. The shiitake helps to dissolve fat and protein deposits, while the kombu gives minerals and counters the weakening effect of the daikon and shiitake.

FOOT BATH

The Foot Bath helps stimulate blood and energy flow and to warm the body. It is good for kidney weakness and for insomnia. It is best done before bedtime.

1.   Place a handful of any kind of sea salt in hot water (salt may be eliminated for certain conditions.)

2.   Immerse feet ankle-high into water for 3-5 minutes.

GINGER BODY SCRUB

This is similar to the Body Scrub, but stronger. The purpose is to promote better circulation and energy flow through the entire body.

1. Heat about one gallon of water until it is hot but not boiling.

2. Meanwhile, grate enough ginger root to equal the size of a small baseball.

3. When the water becomes hot, reduce heat to low, and place the ginger into a single layer of cheesecloth. Tie with a string and squeeze the ginger juice from the cheesecloth sack into the water. (The water at this point should be just below the boiling point.)

4. Place the sack into the pot and allow it to steep in the water without boiling for about five minutes.

5. Dip a small cotton towel or cloth in hot water. Wring out the excess water.

6. Scrub the whole body, dipping the towel or cloth into hot water again when cool. Be sure to include the hands and feet and each finger and toe.

7. The skin should become pink or slightly red. This result may take a few days to achieve, if the skin is clogged with accumulated fats.

Note: • Water left over from a Ginger Compress may be used for a Body Scrub.

GINGER COMPRESS

The purpose of the Ginger Compress is to dissolve stagnation and tension, melt blockages, and stimulate blood circulation and energy flow.

1. Heat about one gallon of water, but do not bring to a boil.

2. Meanwhile, grate enough ginger root to equal the size of a small baseball.

3. When the water becomes hot, reduce heat to low, and place the ginger into a single layer of cheesecloth. Tie with a string and squeeze the ginger juice from the cheesecloth sack into the water. (The water at this point should be just below the boiling point. Also the string should be long enough so that the other end hangs out of the pot for easy retrieval.)

4. Place the sack into the pot and allow it to steep in the water without boiling for about five minutes.

5. Dip a towel into the ginger water, wring out tightly (using a long wooden cooking spoon or stick), and apply it to the desired area on the body. Cover with a second dry towel to hold in the heat.

6. Change the towel every two to three minutes, replacing it with a fresh hot towel. This can be done by using two towels and alternating them so that the skin does not cool off between applications.

7. Continue the applications for about 10 to 15 minutes or until the area becomes pink.

Notes: • Be sure to keep the towels even on the back, not turned up at one or both ends. It is better to keep the pot on the flame in between applications of towels, so that the water remains consistently hot, rather than turn off the flame or place the pot on the floor next to the person.

• The Ginger Compress is not recommended for use on the brain or on the head when high fever is present, on the lower abdominal area during pregnancy, for appendicitis, or for a baby or an older person.

• For cancer, this remedy is often used preceding a Taro Potato Plaster or other plaster. But do not use a Ginger Compress in this case more than once or twice, and for no more than a total duration of 3 to 5 minutes for each towel.

GREEN CLAY PLASTER

Clay has been used traditionally all around the world to draw out excess fluid and fat, to provide relief from aches and pains in the joints, and to help reduce any accumulation of fat. Green clay is available in many natural foods stores.

1.   Mix green clay with enough water to make into a sticky paste.

2.   Apply paste directly onto affected area and cover with a cotton towel.

3.   Leave on three hours or overnight.

HOT OR COLD TOWEL COMPRESS

Hot towels can be used to relieve tension and reduce pain, especially on areas of the body that are tight from overconsumption of animal food, salt, or other more extreme yang foods. For example, a headache in the back of the head is usually caused by these foods, and applying a hot towel will help ease the ache.

Cold towels can be used to relieve tension and reduce pain caused by too much sugar, sweets, soft drinks, fruit, ice cream, and other more extreme yin foods. For example, a headache in the front of the head is usually caused by these type of foods, and applying a cold towel will help ease the ache.

In some cases, hot and cold towels may be alternated every few minutes. For example, leg cramps (usually caused by extreme yin foods, but characterized by yang cramping) can be treated in this way. First massage towards and immediately above the cramping region (but not on it directly). Then apply alternately towels drenched in hot and cold water.

1. Dip plain, cotton towels in hot or cold water and apply to affected area.

2. Remove towels as they lose their strength, replacing them with fresh towels for up to 7 minutes or until area becomes pink.

KOMBU PLASTER

Kombu is a sea vegetable that is used daily in macrobiotic cooking. It also has many medicinal applications and is used in teas and plasters. This remedy is good for burns from radiation (such as medical X-rays), skin lesions, and scars. It is also good to help relieve stagnation and tumors caused by dairy consumption.

1. Soak strips of kombu (the length depends on the area to be covered) and cut to proper size, enough for a double layer.

2. Apply the soaked kombu to the affected area, directly on the skin, in double layers.

3. Cover with a cotton cloth and leave on for three hours or longer. The cloth or towels help to soften the kombu prior to removing.

KOMBU TEA

This tea is good for strengthening the blood. It helps to discharge animal fats and proteins from the body. Traditionally known for its calming properties, it aids in restoring the nervous function and in promoting clear thinking.

1. Wipe off a three-inch piece of dry kombu with a wet cloth.

2. Place the kombu in one quart of water and bring to a boil.

3. Reduce the heat and simmer gently (covered with a lid) until the quantity of water is reduced by half (about 10 to 15 minutes).

4. Drink one cup while hot. You may reheat the remaining tea and drink up to 2 or 3 cups a day.

KUZU DRINKS

Kuzu is a plant or vine that has big roots and is traditionally dug out toward winter, washed in a cold stream, peeled, chopped, dried, washed again, dried again, etc. and made into a powder. Originally kuzu came from Orient, and about one hundred years ago it was brought to the West in a trade fair between the U.S. and Japan. The U.S. government asked the visiting Japanese if they knew of some plant to strengthen riverbanks and they suggested kuzu. Kuzu adapted very well, especially in Georgia, South Carolina, and the southern states. Today, however, it is the #1 headache in those regions and is known as *kudzu*. It is so strong that it has taken over whole fields, parking lots, shopping malls, and other areas.

In macrobiotic cooking, we use kuzu as a thickener to make wonderful sauces, gravies, puddings, and other dishes. We also use it in many home remedies. Kuzu is not too hot or cold, too yin or yang. It makes body temperature and metabolism even. We can make a kuzu drink more yin or yang by adding a pungent or salty taste. All organs of the body are helped by kuzu. It has a neutralizing effect.

In the Far East today, potato starch or white rice powder is added to modern remedies instead of kuzu because the price is lower. Oriental food stores here are selling this kuzu substitute, but we get worse if we use that one. American kuzu is a big treasure. I hope our friends here will develop kuzu or kudzu into a natural foods industry. Rather than be regarded as a nuisance, it can help feed and heal the world.

• See Ame-Kuzu
• See Ume-Sho Kuzu Tea

LEAFY GREENS JUICE

This special drink was originally devised to treat liver disorders, especially yang conditions resulting from eating eggs. It helps to dissolve heavy, stagnated protein, animal fat, and cholesterol deposits. To obtain counterbalancing, light, upward energy from leafy greens, it is easier for many people to take the juice of young barley plants (sold under the name Green Magma in the natural foods store) or another preparation, but this is not as effective. This drink may be taken daily.

1. Very finely chop two or three kinds of large leafy green vegetables (kale, collards, dandelion, daikon or turnip leaves, or Chinese cabbage).

2. Add twice the amount of cold water.

3. Bring to a gentle boil and simmer for 3 to 5 minutes.

4. Strain out the solid vegetables.

5. Add a pinch of sea salt or a few drops of shoyu/soy sauce toward the end of simmering and stir.

6. Drink hot or at room temperature.

Note: • You may or may not reuse the leafy green vegetables.

Variation: • Heat one cup fresh celery or leafy green vegetable juice; add a small pinch of sea salt. Simmer for three to five minutes. Drink hot, warm, or at room temperature.

LOTUS ROOT AND GINGER PLASTER

Lotus root—the long, many chambered, pale root of the lotus plant—is known traditionally for helping to dissolve excess mucus in the lungs, bronchi, throat, or sinuses. This is often caused by dairy food consumption, but lotus is good to release any kind of stagnation, such as that from chicken and egg fat, as well.

This remedy is traditionally known for its effectiveness in dispersing and moving stagnated mucus in the respiratory system. Activate the area to be treated first with a hot towel or Ginger Compress for 5 minutes. Generally stagnation begins to loosen up and mucus starts to drain within three applications of this plaster. Calcified stones in the sinuses sometimes are loosened and come out with sneezing. Stubborn ones can take three weeks to discharge.

1.   Grate enough fresh lotus root to cover the area about one-half inch thick.

2.   Mix thoroughly with 5 percent grated ginger and 10-15 percent unbleached white flour.

3.   Spread the mixture on a cloth or paper towel and apply directly to the skin (not the cloth side).

4.   Leave on for 20 minutes to one hour.

Notes: • To dissolve mucus deposits in the sinuses, you may leave the plaster on for several hours or overnight. In this case, sew a gauze mask with holes for the nose and eyes. Lotus plaster should cover the area around the eyes and above the nose. This application should be repeated for 7 to 10 days, and may sometimes take up to 2 or 3 weeks to the sinuses. Watery or thick mucus may start to be discharged form the eyes and nose.

LOTUS ROOT TEA

This tea is good to relieve lung congestion, clear up sinus problems, and ease chronic coughing.

Usually, salt is used for seasoning with this drink. Since its purpose is to take out or neutralize excessive protein, we don't use shoyu as that has protein. Also the tea is sweeter with salt.

This tea is most effective when prepared from fresh lotus root. However, if fresh is not available, you may use dried lotus root or lotus root powder.

With fresh lotus root:

1. Wash the root and grate one-half cup. Place the pulp in a piece of cheesecloth and squeeze out the juice. (The pulp may be saved and added to other dishes.)

2. Place the juice in a saucepan with an equal amount of water. Add a pinch of sea salt or a few drops of shoyu/soy sauce.

3. Bring to a boil and let simmer gently on a low flame for 2-3 minutes. Drink this tea, which should be thick and creamy, while hot. You may also add a few drops of grated ginger juice toward the end, if your condition permits.

With dried lotus root:

1. Place one-third ounce (about 10 grams) of dried lotus root in one cup of water. Let it sit for a few minutes until soft, then chop finely. Mash in a suribachi.

2. Return the finely chopped lotus root to the soaking water. Add a pinch of sea salt or a few drops of shoyu/soy sauce.

3. Bring to a boil and allow to simmer gently for approximately 15 minutes.

4. Strain the liquid and drink while hot. You may also add a few drops of grated ginger juice toward the end, if your condition permits.

5. You may use the pulp in other dishes.

With lotus root powder:

1. Use one teaspoon of lotus root powder per person and per serving. Add one cup of cold water per teaspoon of powder and stir to dissolve.

2. Add a pinch of sea salt or a few drops of shoyu/soy sauce. You may also add a couple of drops of grated ginger juice, if your condition permits.

3. Heat on a low flame but do not boil. Turn off the heat when the liquid begins to simmer. Drink while hot.

LOTUS ROOT AND SHIITAKE TEA

This tea is helpful to decompose heavy animal-quality fat and mucus.

1. Soak a one to one-half inch diameter dried shiitake mushroom. Chop or finely slice when soft.

2. Follow the same steps as in the previous recipe with fresh or dried lotus root.

3. Add two cups water (you may include the soaking water from the shiitake mushroom).

4. Bring to a boil, reduce the flame and simmer for approximately 7 to 10 minutes. Add a pinch of sea salt or shoyu/soy sauce toward the end. Drink while hot.

Note: • Donko shiitakes are the highest grade shiitake mushroom.

MISO PLASTER

Soybeans have a cooling effect on the body. Raw soybeans soaked in water, crushed, and applied on the affected area can take out fever.

Miso—the fermented soybean paste used daily in macrobiotic cooking for soup, condiments, and seasoning—also has many medicinal applications. A Miso Plaster consists of raw miso applied directly on the body.

It is good for burns, including those from radiation. It is good for cuts and will stop bleeding, but should not be used for puncture wounds. The enzymes in miso neutralize bacteria and help to prevent infection. In the kitchen, nicks and cuts when cutting vegetables can be treated with a dab of miso on the hand or finger.

A Miso Plaster can also draw out bee stingers, help relieve itchy skin diseases, and reduce any kind of swelling. It is an essential ingredient in a home first-aid kit. Use regular barley, rice, or hatcho miso for this purpose. It is all right if the miso has been pasteurized. It will still be effective.

1. Place raw miso over the affected area, about one quarter to one half inch thick.

2. Wrap with a single layer of cheesecloth.

Note: • **When putting miso directly on the skin, do not pack it down firmly, as this can cause scarring.**

Variation: • See Brown Rice/Miso Plaster.

MOXA

Moxabustion (or moxa) is a traditional Far Eastern healing method that employs heat along the meridians and points to activate and supply energy to specific regions, organs, systems, and functions of the body. Moxa can be used for general strengthening, such as on Stomach Meridian Point 36 on the leg for health and longevity; to help relieve specific symptoms such as constipation or facial problems, e.g., Large Intestine Point 4 on the hand; or for chronic conditions such as multiple sclerosis, on certain points along the spine. It has also been used for acute symptoms, such as food poisoning, and for helping someone who is dying recover strength, energy, or consciousness.

Traditionally, dried mugwort is used, and long sticks of moxa or small moxa cones are available in acupuncture clinics, Oriental markets, or, occasionally, natural foods stores.

1. To apply, light the moxa stick and approach the point in a slow, gentle clockwise spiral.

2. Hold moxa stick above the point (not touching the skin) for several seconds until the person feels strong heat.

3. Then pull back the stick and after a few seconds apply again in the same way. Usually five times is enough for most applications, though emergency treatments may take more time.

Note: • Locations of the points are different for everyone. So you can't just mechanically follow an acupuncture chart or diagram in a book. **A thorough understanding of Far Eastern philosophy and medicine, including the meridian system, is recommended before use of this method. Moxa is generally not used for yang conditions or symptoms characterized by excess energy.**

Variation: • If a moxa stick is not available, an ordinary cigarette may be used.

MU TEA

This tea was developed by George Ohsawa. He modified a
traditional herbal remedy called *Chujo-to*, "Hot Drink," which was
invented over 300-400 years ago. It was used to strengthen
women's reproductive organs and was very popular. George
Ohsawa slightly changed it, and it is good for everyone. *Mu* means
"nothing," and comes from a phrase "mu cha kui cha." *Mu cha*
refers to confusion, disorder, mixed up theories, while *kui* means
nine. George took the name Mu Tea Nine Herbs and used nine
ingredients, including ginseng.

Ordinarily, in the macrobiotic way of eating, we do not use
ginseng, because it is is very yang and gives constricting effects.
Breathing becomes difficult and body temperature becomes cold.
However, by blending it with more yin herbs, the effect is
neutralized. Still, Mu Tea is a slightly yang drink, and it is better not
to cook it or rewarm it a long time or strong effects may come. In
addition to the Mu Tea with nine herbs, there is another variety with
sixteen herbs, that is even slightly more yang.

Mu Tea is good to help relieve swelling, inflammations,
weakness in sexual organs; wet mucousy coughs and respiratory
disorders; and swollen intestines. It can help relieve tiredness and is
helpful for losing weight. Take several times a week for 3 to 4
weeks.

1.   For healthy persons, boil a tea bag for 10 minutes in 3 cups
        of water.

2.   For persons with yin conditions such as a weak stomach,
        yin coughing, menstrual cramps or irregular menstruation,
        boil in 3 cups of water for 5 minutes, then let simmer for 25
        minutes or until only half the liquid (1 1/2 cups) remains.

MUSTARD PLASTER

The Mustard Plaster dissolves stagnation and stimulates circulation, especially in the lungs. It can help relieve mucous accumulation or coughing and is good for muscle stiffness. It is a traditional Far Eastern remedy and I received it as a child.

1. While preparing the plaster, warm up two towels.

2. Crush enough mustard seeds to obtain a handful of mustard powder. You may also use mustard powder or, if unavailable, mustard spread from a jar.

3. Bring some water to a boil and add enough to the mustard to make a moist paste. The consistency should be light and soft, something like mustard from a jar.

4. Spread the paste onto one-half of a triple layer of paper towels or one layer of waxed paper. (The area should be large enough to cover the chest if it is being used for the lungs or upper back.) Fold in half to cover the paste on both sides.

5. Spread a towel on the area to be treated. Place the mixture in this wrapper of paper towels or waxed paper on top of the towel and cover with the second towel.

6. Leave the plaster on until the heat starts to feel uncomfortable, usually 10 to 15 minutes.

Notes: • The skin will become red, which is normal. The effects will last as long as the red color remains.

• **Do not apply mustard directly on the skin as it will burn.**

• When using this plaster on children, mix in an equal amount of flour.

• If some mustard inadvertently leaks and burns the skin, spread a small amount of olive oil or other light vegetable quality oil on the affected area.

• For lung troubles, you may apply the plaster on the chest, back, or both.

• In case of an acute condition, you may apply the plaster 2 or 3 times a day, but please refrain from too frequent use as it may burn the skin if repeated too often.

PEARL BARLEY PLASTER

Pearl barley, also called *hato mugi* or Job's Tears, is a grass, not a grain. We use it in macrobiotic cooking as an occasional supplement or replacement for ordinary barley. (Do not confuse *pearl* barley with *pearled* barley, or hulled barley. Pearl barley has a distinctive black spot or dot on one end.)

In Far Eastern medicine, pearl barley has traditionally been used to melt excess animal protein and fat and to beautify the skin. This plaster is good for harmonizing body energy and drawing out and softening excess fat or protein. It is especially good for clearing up moles, warts, and boils.

1. Cook pearl barley to a soft consistency, using one part grain to three parts water. Let the grain cool to room temperature.

2. Mash cooked grain in a suribachi until it becomes a paste.

3. Add 5 percent grated ginger a little white flour. Mix thoroughly.

4. Spread the mixture from one-half to one-inch thick on a cotton cloth.

5. Apply the mixture directly to affected area (not the cloth side). Secure it in place with a bandage or tie with a cotton strip. Leave on for several hours or overnight.

Variation: • Add from one-third to two-thirds cup fresh, chopped and mashed green cabbage or other leafy greens to the above mixture.

POTATO AND CABBAGE PLASTER

This plaster may be used when taro potato is not available for the Taro Potato Plaster or when regular potato is specifically recommended. It has a softening and drawing effect on tumors.

1. Grate potato (green potatoes are best).

2. If the potato is very watery, place it in a double layer of cheesecloth, and squeeze out the excess water before combining it with the other ingredients.

3. Mash equal amount of finely chopped raw leafy greens in a suribachi (kale, collards, watercress, etc.).

4. Add about 10 percent grated ginger to the mixture and mix well.

5. If the paste is still too watery, add some unbleached white flour to thicken it to the consistency of mud or wet cement.

6. Spread the mixture about one-half inch thick on a clean cotton cloth.

7. Apply the mixture directly on the infected area. Leave the plaster on for about four hours.

RANSHO (RAW EGG AND SHOYU/SOY SAUCE)

Ordinarily we don't eat eggs in the standard macrobiotic way of eating. However, for certain medicinal conditions, egg may be beneficial. *Ransho* (a combination of raw egg and shoyu or natural soy sauce) strengthens the heart quickly. The purpose of the egg is to provide a large volume of shoyu and enable the body to absorb it rapidly.

During sports competitions in the Orient, mothers traditionally used to give Ransho to their children to make their hearts strong. But people in those days were not eating much animal food, so they could take this strong combination. For vegetarians it is good, but for people eating animal food it has such a powerful effect that it is better not given.

Ransho has been used to activate the heart, especially for heart failure caused by more yin factors such as sugar, sweets, soft drinks, alcohol, and other extremely expansive foods. For yang heart failure, such as that caused by meat, poultry, eggs, cheese, or too much salt, Ransho has the opposite effect and makes the condition worse.

To tell if a heart attack or stroke is caused by more yin or yang, look at the person's hands after the attack. If open, the cause is more yin and Ransho can be given. If the hands are closed, it is more yang and Ransho should not be given. Instead, give a yang person apple juice or something more yin.

If you can't decide whether it is yin or yang, put a raw egg in miso soup with plenty of scallions, Chinese cabbage, onions, and a little ginger. That will make the heart beat actively and improve circulation. This is also good for severe anemia.

1. Break egg and beat yolk and white together. Use an organic, fertilized egg if possible.

2 Add 1 tablespoon of shoyu (natural soy sauce) to egg.

3. Mix together very, very well, beating for several minutes.

4   Give only once the first day, and then, if needed, a second time a half day or day later, but no more than twice altogether.

Variation: • For ordinary, milder use, use the raw egg and shoyu as is. For a stronger effect, use just the egg yolk and shoyu.

• The traditional way of measuring was to take one of the shells of the broken egg and fill it half full with shoyu.

Notes: **• Ransio is good for yin conditions—such as someone near death—to make the heart start beating. In this case, give teaspoon by teaspoon, repeating two or three times a day if necessary. But be very careful; in other cases, such as a drug overdose which is also caused by extreme yin. Giving Ransho may produce the opposite effect and cause the heart to stop. In the case of a drug overdose, yin should be dispersed by giving strong miso soup with ginger. This is much safer. Ideally, give Ransho under the supervision of an experienced macrobiotic teacher.**

• For emergency first aid in case of a heart attack or stroke, press, bite, or apply fire (moxa) to the little finger to activate the heart. The heart meridian ends just below the nail on the inside of the little fingers and stimulation here will help revive the person. Or put strong pressure on the nails of the little finger with a needle, chopstick, or finger pressure. Press the heart point on the lower inside of the wrists to activate the heart meridian, especially on the left side. Breathe strongly while pressing. Repeat several times for up to several minutes or until the person begins to stabilize.

RICE BRAN PLASTER

Generally, commercial soaps, creams, and lotions clog the meridians, holes, and sweat glands, impeding ki flow. People who eat dairy food are especially attracted to these products. Dry skin comes from a layer of oil and fat blocking the skin, not from a lack of oil.

Rice bran is very helpful for this condition. Rice bran is also good for all diseases of the skin, including allergies, boils, poison ivy, rashes, infections, and a red or purplish color. Rice bran is also good for candida and yeast infections, inflammations, and soothing broken bones. It may also be put on the toes for frostbite lesions.

Traditionally, rice bran (known as *nuka* in the East) has been used for thousands of years. Rice was traditionally kept unhulled until eaten and then the polishings, or *bran*, was kept for pickling and soap. Nuka will make the skin very clean and shiny. It has strong healing power.

1. To a handful of rice bran, add about one third as much flour, and mix. Use rice flour if available or hato mugi flour. Otherwise you may use wheat or white flour.

2. Add cold water as needed to make a thick paste.

3. Put mixture in a cheesecloth, dip in hot water, and apply on the skin. Rinse plaster off and apply a fresh one when it becomes warm.

Note: • Nuka water can be applied around the vagina, but do not use as a douche because the brany texture may be irritating to this region. Nuka may also be added to the bath.

Variation: • Use wheat or oat bran if rice bran is not available.

SALT PACK

The purpose of the Salt Pack is to heat and ease the tension in various parts of the body, including stiff muscles, the abdominal area in case of diarrhea, menstrual or intestinal cramps, and stomach cramps.

1. Dry-roast one and one-half pound of any kind of sea salt in a stainless steel skillet until it is very hot.

2. Wrap the hot salt in a thick cotton towel and tie securely with a string.

3. Apply to the affected area.

4. Change the salt or reheat when it starts to cool off.

5. Save the salt as it can be used for a salt pack again. Eventually discard when the salt becomes gray and no longer holds heat.

Note: • Sand may be used, if salt is not readily available.

SEA VEGETABLE DOUCHE

This remedy helps to eliminate stagnated mucus and fat in the region of the uterus, vagina, or cervix, especially that caused by dairy, sugar, or chocolate. It is especially recommended for middle-aged or older women or for anyone who has consumed a lot of dairy food. Do daily for about 10 days.

1. Add one 5-inch strip of kombu and 1 to 2 umeboshi plums to one quart of cold water.

2. Bring to a gentle boil; cover; lower flame.

3. Simmer 20 minutes, then strain out plums and kombu.

4. Allow to cool to body temperature before douching.

SESAME-GINGER OIL

In the Far East, sesame seeds were considered medicine for longevity. By adding a little ginger oil to the sesame, we can increase its effectiveness. This remedy is good for arthritis, rheumatism, or any pain in the joints or to activate blood circulation. It is good for dandruff and for hair falling out. It can also be put in the ear or eye (see note below). Use toasted dark sesame oil if available. Otherwise, light sesame is suitable.

1. Grate fresh ginger root and press out 1 teaspoon of juice from the gratings.

2. Mix with an equal amount of sesame oil.

3. Shake well before using and apply to the affected region for 5 to 10 minutes.

Notes: • If burning sensation results, reduce the ginger.

• If put in the eye, first heat the oil, let cool, and strain through a handerchief.

SESAME SEED TEA

This remedy is good to loosen digestive stagnation and relieve constipation. It is also good to grow and darken the hair, to relieve troubled eyes, promote breast milk production, and treat menstrual irregularity. Use black sesame seeds if available. Otherwise, use white (tan or brown) ones.

1. To 2 tablespoons of sesame seeds, slightly crushed, add 1 cup of boiling water and cook 15 minutes. Drink the seeds as well as the liquid.

Variation: • A sweet taste, such as barley malt, may be added if desired. This is particularly helpful in stimulating hair growth. Take daily for 2 to 3 weeks.

SHIITAKE MUSHROOM TEA

Traditionally this tea was known to reduce fever, to help dissolve animal-quality fat, and to help relax a contracted or tense condition. Dried shiitake mushrooms are preferred to fresh whenever possible.

1. Soak one shiitake mushroom in one cup of water for 20-30 minutes.

2. When shiitake mushroom is soft, finely chop.

3. Bring to a boil. Reduce flame and simmer gently for 10 to 15 minutes.

4. Add a pinch of sea salt or a few drops of shoyu/soy sauce toward the end. Drink while hot.

Note: • For children one year old or under, do not add any seasoning to the tea.

SHOYU/SOY SAUCE BANCHA TEA

This drink is good to strengthen the blood if an overly acidic condition exists; to relieve fatigue; to relieve headaches due to the overconsumption of simple sugars and/or fruit juice; and to stimulate good blood circulation.

1. Place up to one teaspoon of shoyu/soy sauce in a tea cup and pour in hot bancha twig or stem tea.

2. Stir and drink while hot.

Note: • Be careful to pour the hot tea over the shoyu in a cup, not the other way around (adding the shoyu to the pot).

SWEET VEGETABLE DRINK

Several years ago, I developed this drink to help offset the effects of chicken, egg, and cheese consumption, leading to hypoglycemia, or chronic low blood sugar, a condition that affects about 75 or 80 percent of everyone in modern society.

Sweet Vegetable Drink is good for softening tightness caused by heavy animal food consumption and for relaxing the body and muscles. It is especially beneficial for softening the pancreas and helping to stabilize blood sugar levels. A small cup may be taken daily or every other day, especially in the mid to late afternoon. It will satisfy the desire for a sweet taste and help reduce cravings for simple sugars and other stronger sweets.

1.   Use equal amounts of four sweet vegetables, finely chopped (onions, carrots, cabbage, and sweet winter squash).

2.   Boil four times the amount of water, add chopped vegetables and allow to boil, uncovered, for 2 to 3 minutes. Reduce flame to low, cover, and let simmer for 20 minutes.

3.   Strain the vegetables from the broth. (You may occasionally use them later in soups and stews).

4.   Drink the broth, either hot or at room temperature.

Notes: • No seasoning is used in this recipe.

• Sweet vegetable broth may be kept in the refrigerator for up to two days, but should be warmed again or allowed to return to room temperature before drinking.

Variation: • Substitute daikon and lotus root for carrots and squash; prepare according to recipe above.

TARO POTATO PLASTER

Taro is a small, hairy tuber native to Hawaii, the Caribbean, Southeast Asia, and other tropical and semitropical regions. It is used in cooking in these regions as well as medicinally.

Traditionally, the Taro Potato Plaster has been used to draw out blood, pus, carbon, and excess protein and fat from boils and tumors. Dr. Sagen Ishizuka, the grandfather of modern macrobiotics in Japan, used this remedy for tumors caused by egg, fish, or other animal food consumption, and George Ohsawa received it from him. It is good for strong yang conditions such as colon, pancreas, or liver tumors, but for yin type conditions such as breast cancer it can cause the tumor to spread. It is also better to put the Taro Plaster on isolated organs and not on the prostate, ovaries, or other organs which (though yang) are located close to other organs and which might cause the tumor to spread.

Before applying the Taro Potato Plaster, you may do a very short-time Ginger Compress (3 to 5 minutes) to warm up the skin and to increase the effectiveness of the plaster.

If the plaster feels too cold, a salt pack may be placed on top.

If plaster feels itchy, you may rub sesame oil on the skin before the plaster is applied the next time.

1. Remove the skin from the taro potato and grate the potato.

2. Add 5 percent grated ginger and mix. (If the paste causes too much itching, you may omit the ginger.)

3. If the paste is very wet, add a little unbleached white flour for finer consistency. The paste, however, should remain moist and have the consistency of wet cement or mud.

4. Spread the mixture about one-half inch thick on a clean cotton cloth.

5. Apply the mixture directly on the infected area (not the cloth side). Leave the plaster on for about four hours.

6. If the plaster has dried and is difficult or painful to remove, apply enough warm water to moisten the paste.

Note: • **For cancer or other serious illness, it is recommended that you see a qualified macrobiotic teacher regarding the use of this plaster. It is not recommended for malignancies of the breast, spine, reproductive organs, and other areas of the body.**

TOFU PLASTER

The Tofu Plaster is good to help relieve inflammations, swellings, fevers, burns, dental abcesses, and bruises. The tofu is cold and therefore makes yang or contraction, serving to neutralize heat or inflammation. It is more effective than ice.

This remedy has been successfully used in some cases of paralysis, such as stroke, or for a concussion such as a motocycle accident in which the person is left unconscious. In such a case, after seeking medical attention and going to the hospital, immediately apply crushed, cold tofu to the affected part of the head, and continuously make and apply Tofu Plasters. They will help to heal and repair the damage quickly. Apply as soon as possible. Four hours later may be too late.

1.   Squeeze out the liquid from a block of tofu and mash tofu in a suribachi. Mix well to take out all lumps.

2.   Add 10-20 percent unbleached white flour and 5 percent grated ginger. Mix well. (It is better to peel the ginger before grating for cool plasters as ginger can irritate the skin.)

3.   Apply the mixture (which should be moist) directly to the skin and cover with a towel. You may want to secure it in place with a bandage, or tie with a cotton strip.

4.   Change the plaster every 2 to 3 hours, or when it becomes hot.

Variation: • Tofu plaster may be combined with chopped, mashed leafy greens (as in the Chlorophyll Plaster), especially for hemorrhages.

• A Tofu and Grain Plaster may be used as an alternative, especially if the Tofu Plaster feels too cold. Make by mixing 50 percent cooked whole grain (rice or barley) which has cooled to room temperature with 50 percent squeezed and mashed tofu.

UME-SHO BANCHA

Umeboshi—dried, salted plums— are widely used in macrobiotic cooking and home remedies. The ume plums are especially aged and contain a balance of energy that neutralizes extremes of both yin and yang.

This drink is good to strengthen the blood; to regulate digestion and circulation; to relieve fatigue and weakness; and to obtain relief from an overconsumption of simple sugars, fruit, fruit juices, or acid-forming foods or beverages.

1. Place one-half or one umeboshi plum in a tea cup with one-half or one teaspoon of shoyu/soy sauce.

2. Pour in hot bancha stem or twig tea and stir well. Drink hot, eating the plum.

Note: • The strongest, most effective umeboshi plums for medicinal use are aged 5 years and are presently available in limited supply from the Kushi Foundation Store in Becket.

UME-SHO KUZU DRINK

This drink is good to strengthen and promote good digestion and restore energy.

1. Dissolve one heaping teaspoon of kuzu in 2 or 3 tablespoons of cold water.

2. Add one cup cold water to the dissolved kuzu.

3. Add the pulp of one-half to one umeboshi plum that has been chopped and ground to a paste.

4. Bring to a boil over a medium flame, stirring constantly to avoid lumping, until the liquid becomes translucent. Reduce the flame as low as possible.

5. Add from several drops to one-half teaspoon of shoyu/soy sauce and stir gently. Simmer for 2 to 3 minutes. Drink while hot.

UME-SHO KUZU WITH GINGER

For the same purposes as Ume-Sho Kuzu Drink but more efficient for promoting digestion and for stimulating body warmth.

1. Prepare in the same manner as above, but add one-eighth teaspoon fresh grated ginger toward the end and stir gently.

2. Simmer for one-half minute and drink while hot.

UMEBOSHI TEA

This is a very refreshing and cooling drink for the summer.

1.　　Simmer the pulp of one umeboshi for one-half hour in a quart of water in a covered saucepan.

2.　　Strain and, if necessary, dilute with more water. Allow to cool before drinking.

APPENDIX

THE STANDARD
MACROBIOTIC DIET*

Daily Foods

Whole Cereal Grains
On the average, 50 percent of daily intake by weight should include cooked, organically grown, whole cereal grains, which may be prepared in a variety of ways. These include brown rice, millet, oats, corn, rye, wheat, buckwheat, and others. A portion of this amount may consist of noodles or pasta, unyeasted whole grain breads, and other partially processed grains or grain products. However, whole grain prepared in whole form should ideally form the center of every meal.

Soups
About 5 to 10 percent of our daily food (1 to 2 cups or bowls) may include soup made with vegetables, sea vegetables (such as wakame or kombu), grains, or beans. Seasonings include miso, shoyu (natural soy sauce), and sea salt. The flavor should not be too salty and should be suitable to personal condition and taste.

Vegetables
About 25 to 30 percent of our daily food consists of vegetables, locally and organically grown whenever possible. As examples, vegetables for daily use include: green leafy vegetables: bok choy, Chinese cabbage, collard greens, kale, leeks, mustard greens, parsley, scallions, turnip greens, and watercress. Round vegetables: acorn squash, broccoli, Brussel sprouts, butternut squash, buttercup squash, cabbage, cauliflower, onions, pumpkin, rutabaga, and turnip. Root vegetables: burdock, carrots, daikon, lotus root, parsnips, and radish. Vegetables may be cooked in various styles: steaming, boiling, sautéed with a small

---

* Guidelines are the standard average in a temperate climate zone. For tropical or polar (cold climate) guidelines, please see *Standard Macrobiotic Diet* by Michio Kushi (One Peaceful World Press).

amount of sesame oil, and occasionally deep-fried or baked as health permits. A small portion may be eaten occasionally as fresh raw salad and frequently as boiled or pressed salad.

Beans and Sea Vegetables

About 5 to 10 percent of daily diet incudes cooked beans and sea vegetables. The most suitable beans for day to day use are azuki beans, chickpeas, and lentils. Other beans may be used on occasion. Bean products such as tofu, tempeh, and natto may be used daily. Sea vegetables such as nori, wakame, and kombu are recommended for daily use. Hiziki and arame may be taken two or three times a week as a small side dish. All others may be used occasionally as desired. Sea vegetables may be prepared in a variety of ways: cooked with beans or vegetables, used in soups or served as side dishes, or flavored with a moderate amount of shoyu, sea salt, umeboshi plum, or other seasoning.

Seasonings

Seasonings are used to enhance flavor and taste and are recommended for use in moderate amounts. Seasonings to be used daily include unrefined white sea salt with a balanced mineral content, traditionally made miso that has aged two or more years, and natural shoyu. They should be cooked with the foods, not added at the table. Cooking oil should be vegetable quality only, especially unrefined sesame oil (light or dark) or unrefined corn oil.

Condiments

Condiments allow for individual variety and taste. They are kept on the table and used, if desired, in small amounts. Recommended condiments include gomashio (sesame salt usually made from 1 part roasted sea salt to 16 to 18 parts roasted sesame seeds), umeboshi plums, tekka root vegetable condiment, green nori flakes, and others.

Pickles

A small amount of pickles traditionally made from the highest quality ingredients are eaten daily with meals. A variety of pickles are recommended including sauerkraut, miso pickles, shoyu pickles, and umeboshi pickles.

Beverages

Recommended daily beverages include roasted bancha twig tea (also known as kukicha), roasted brown rice tea, and roasted barley tea. Any traditional tea that does not have an aromatic fragrance or a stimulating effect may be used. For drinking or cooking, good quality water (preferably natural spring or well water) may be used. If these are not available, bottled spring water or filtered tap water are recommended. Avoid excessive liquid consumption and ice cold beverages. Vegetable and fruit juice and good quality beer may be used occasionally as health permits.

Occasional Foods

Fish and Seafood
For people in usual good health, a variety of supplemental foods may be taken. These include fresh low-fat, white-meat fish such as cod, flounder, or sole once or twice a week in modest volume. Fish may be prepared in a variety of ways, especially steaming, boiling, poaching, or lightly sautéing. More fatty red-meat, blue-skinned, and shellfish may be used sparingly as health permits.

Fruit
Fruit, including fresh, dried, and cooked fruits, may be taken two to three times a week. Local and organically grown fruits are prefered, such as apples, cherries, pears, plums, peaches, apricots, berries, and melons. Tropical and semitropical fruits are best avoided in a temperate climate. Frequent use of fruit juice is not advisable. Occasional consumption in warmer weather is suitable as health permits.

Seeds and Nuts
Nuts and seeds such as pumpkin seeds, sesame seeds, sunflower seeds, peanuts, walnuts, and pecans may be enjoyed as a snack. Other snacks include mochi, sushi, rice cakes, and popcorn.

Natural Desserts
Naturally sweetened desserts such as puddings, natural gelatins, cakes, pies, puddings, and cookies may be taken several times a week as health permits. These should be made with good quality ingredients (no eggs, refined flour, or dairy) and naturally sweetened with a grain-based sweetener such as amasake, barley malt, or rice syrup or, occasionally, fruit juice.

Way of Eating

It is important to eat regularly, two to three times a day, and you may eat as much as you want, provided the proportion of daily eating is within suggested guidelines. Please chew thoroughly, and avoid eating three hours before bedtime.

Proper cooking is essential for health. Everyone is encouraged to study cooking. Preparing food in a grateful, loving spirit is very important.

GLOSSARY

Amasake A sweetener or refreshing drink made from sweet brown rice and koji starter that is allowed to ferment into a thick liquid.

Ame A natural sweetener made from rice syrup.

Arame A thin, wiry black sea vegetable.

Azuki A small, dark red bean originally from Japan but also now grown in the United States.

Bancha tea The stems and leaves from mature Japanese tea bushes, also known as kukicha. Bancha tea contains no caffeine.

Brown rice Whole, unpolished rice, containing an ideal balance of minerals, protein, and carbohydrates.

Daikon A long, white radish.

Ginger A spicy, pungent, golden-colored root.

Gomashio Sesame salt made from roasted, ground sesame seeds and sea salt.

Ki Natural electromagnetic energy of heaven and earth that activates the meridians, organs, and tissues of the body.

Kombu A wide, thick, dark green sea vegetable that grows in deep ocean water.

Kuzu A white starch made from the root of a wild plant. Also known as kudzu.

Lotus root The root of water lily, which is brown-skinned with a hollow, chambered, off-white inside.

Meridian A flow of natural electromagnetic energy in the body that activates and charges the organs and functions, tissues and cells.

Miso Fermented soybean paste.

Mochi A rice cake or dumpling made from cooked, pounded sweet rice.

Moxibustion Oriental medical technique of burning mugwort or other herb on the skin to release blocked energy and promote circulation. Also known as Moxa.

Nori Thin sheets of dried sea vegetable, black or dark purple in color when dried, they turn green when roasted over a flame. Used in making vegetable sushi and wrapped around rice balls.

Nuka Rice bran.

Pearl barley A Far Eastern grain-like botanical plant that is also known as hato mugi or Job's Tears.

Sea salt Salt obtained from the ocean and either sun-baked or kiln-baked. Unlike refined table salt, it is high in trace minerals and contains no chemicals, sugar, or other additives.

Shiitake An Oriental mushroom that is now grown in the United States. Scientific name is Lentinus edodes.

Shiso The leaves that are traditionally processed along with umeboshi plums. Also known as beefsteak leaves.

Shoyu Traditional, naturally made soy sauce as distinguished from refined, chemically processed soy sauce.

Suribachi A serrated, glazed clay bowl used with a pestle for grinding and puréing foods and making home remedies.

Taro A potato that has a thick, hairy skin. Also called albi.

Tofu Soybean curd made from soybeans and nigari.

Umeboshi A salty, pickled plum originally from Japan but now also made in the United States. Ume refers to this plum or one of its products.

Yang One of the two complementary and antagonistic forces that combine to produce all phenomena. Yang refers to the relative tendency of contraction, centripetality, fusion, light, density, male, etc. An overly yang condition is reflected in tightness, tension, hardness, dryness, fastness, impatience, and anger.

Yin The antagonistic, complementary force to yang. Yin is the relative tendency of expansion, growth, centrifugality, diffusion, cold, darkness, female, etc. An overly yin condition is reflected in looseness, moistness, memory loss, lack of concentration, slowness, softness, and fragility.

ABOUT THE AUTHOR

Michio Kushi, leader of the international macrobiotic community, was born in Japan in 1926, studied international relations and law at Tokyo University, and came to the United States in 1949. Devoted to the cause of world peace through world health, he and his wife, Aveline, introduced modern macrobiotics to North America. Over the years, he has lectured and given seminars on diet and health, philosophy, and spiritual practice to medical professionals, government officials, and individuals and families around the world, guiding thousands of people to greater health and happiness. Founder and president of the East West Foundation, the Kushi Institute, and One Peaceful World and author of numerous books, he maintains a busy international travel schedule and makes his home in Brookine and Becket, Massachusetts.

Other books by Michio Kushi available from One Peaceful World Press include *Standard Macrobiotic Diet, The Teachings of Michio Kushi, Nine Star Ki, Forgotten Worlds, Healing Harvest, One Peaceful World,* and *The Cancer-Prevention Diet.*

Index